The Magic of Vegetables

Ancient Healing Remedies and Tips

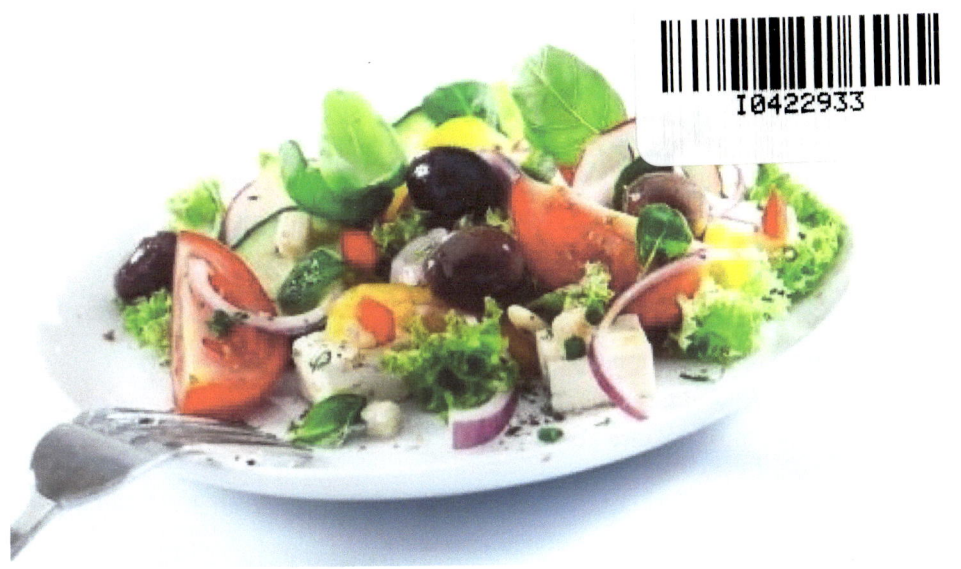

Dueep Jyot Singh

Natural Remedy Series

Mendon Cottage Books

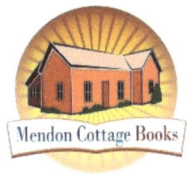

JD-Biz Publishing

Download Free Books!

http://MendonCottageBooks.com

Disclaimer

The information is this book is provided for informational purposes only. It is not intended to be used and medical advice or a substitute for proper medical treatment by a qualified health care provider. The information is believed to be accurate as presented based on research by the author.

The contents have not been evaluated by the U.S. Food and Drug Administration or any other Government or Health Organization and the contents in this book are not to be used to treat cure or prevent disease.

The author or publisher is not responsible for the use or safety of any diet, procedure or treatment mentioned in this book. The author or publisher is not responsible for errors or omissions that may exist.

Warning

The Book is for informational purposes only and before taking on any diet, treatment or medical procedure, it is recommended to consult with your primary health care provider.

Our books are available at

1. Amazon.com
2. Barnes and Noble
3. Itunes
4. Kobo
5. Smashwords
6. Google Play Books

Table of Contents

Introduction

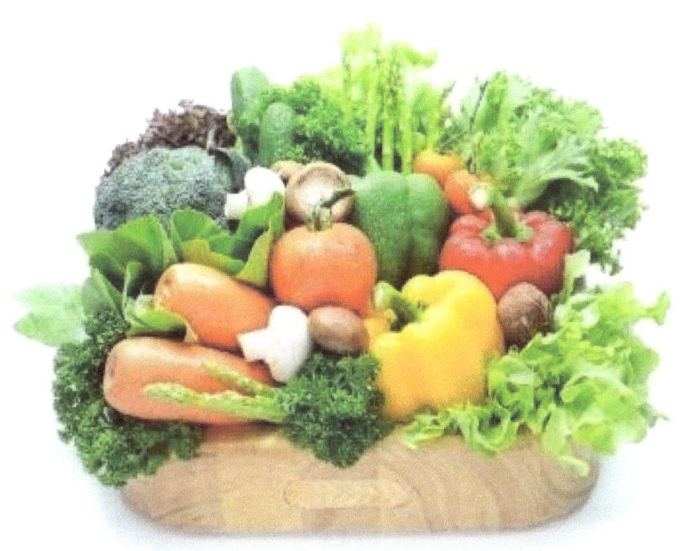

Vegetables are such an integral part of our daily lives, that we really do not bother much about their natural benefits and value. All we know is that they are those greens which we *had to* eat when we were children, because mommy said so, and she was bigger than us. And she was not a good cook. And also, she made every vegetable dish taste so boring, so blah and so bland, that one promised oneself that one would never eat it, when one grew up.

That is the reason why so many of us grow up with an anti-vegetable subconscious feeling. But did you know that these green and leafy vegetables are the reasons why you kept so healthy, so energetic, and so bouncing when you were a kid. They were the natural mineral resources, which provided you with vitamins, minerals, and other essential nutrients, which help your muscles grow healthy, your skin glow and made you look so bright eyed and bushy tailed.

And then you grew up and stopped eating vegetables. Instead, you began eating and other high-protein diet, without any greens or yellows or reds , which were harvested from plants/vines/herbs or shrubs. And that made your body deficient in all the essential vitamins. It also made you less healthy than what you were when you were a kid. And you did not get to know it.

So here are some good reasons why you should eat plant produce, especially when they are green and leafy.

Fibrous, leafy and green vegetables, fresh from the farm are, of course, the pride and joy of every health conscious and proud cook. If the proportions of these vegetables are increased in your daily diet, you are going to lessen your intake of carbohydrates, starch, and grain. This is going to benefit you and the general state of your health in the long run. It also means that you will never suffer from constipation.

Nothing can take the place of cereals and grains in your daily diet in the same manner, vegetables have their own invaluable and irreplaceable place in the diet groups which make up your daily meals.

The benefits of vegetables eaten raw, or cooked, then means that you are going to have a tasty meal, with natural digestive products being added to your system. Your blood circulation is going to get invigorated and your digestive system is going to get rid of any small ailments brought about by eating a starchy, fatty and high-protein high carbohydrate diet.

Vegetables are amazing toxin eliminators. So if you are thinking of detoxifying your body with any star – endorsed detoxifying products, think again. Try increasing the amounts of vegetables in your diet.

The best thing about fibrous vegetables is that it adds the amount of bulk to the fecal material so that it can be eliminated during the regular bowel movements every day. This keeps your system healthy. It also keeps your skin glowing, and you energetic. That is because there are no toxins accumulating in your body and weakening your system.

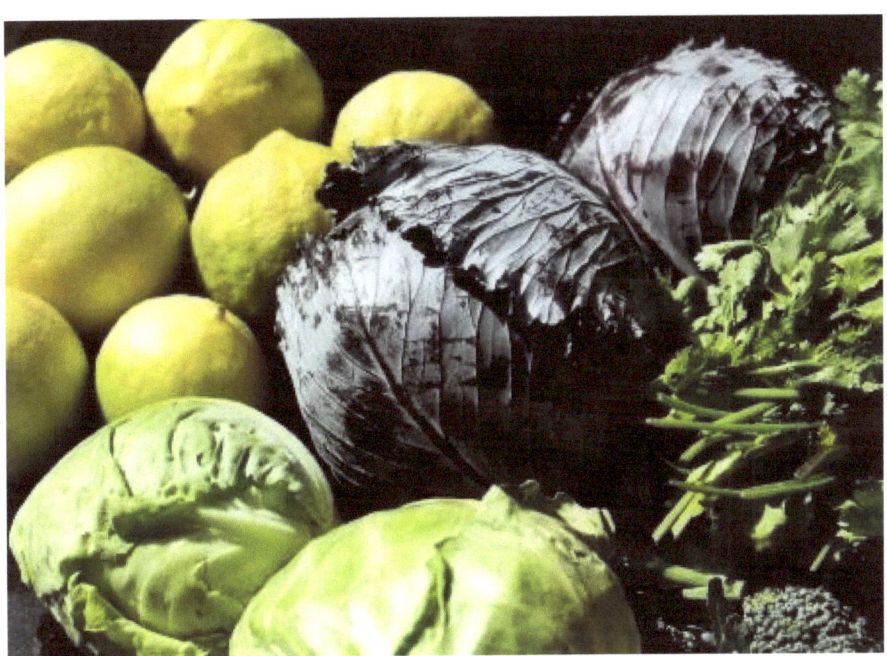

Good to eat, and rich in fiber and other essential nutrients, including vitamins.

These vegetables are best eaten raw – radishes, along with radish leaves, carrots, beetroot and tomatoes. Best eat them, unpeeled. They increase the production of saliva in your mouth. This saliva, when mixed with your food is an extremely important ingredient to aid in digestion.

Also chewing all these vegetables in their raw condition is extremely good exercise for strengthening your teeth, jaws and gums.

You can preserve the green part of the vegetables by wrapping them up in a wet cloth, when you do not have a refrigerator present. But I would suggest using these green leaves as soon as they come in from the market or from your garden instead of waiting for tomorrow.

Do not keep washing them all the time. Scrub and wipe them with a wet cloth, if you have just got them out from the ground, after you had shaken off the dirt. Then leave them in the water for 10 minutes to soak. This is to get rid of all the pesticides. So the soaking in the water is going to get rid of all the pesticides in the leaves. Give the vegetables one last good rinse and scrub and then put them in watertight bags for freezing or for preserving.

You need not wash them again, after you have defrosted them, and when you intend to cook them.

Vegetables should not be overcooked, because this is the easiest way in which you can destroy all their essential mineral nutrients. That is why, vegetables are normally left *al dente* by French and Italians, which means half cooked and a bit difficult to chew. But then, those vegetables are also eaten raw, so one should not worry about their half cooked state.

If you really want those vegetables cooked really well, do not fry them. Instead, steam them, so that their nutrients are not destroyed with powerful heating mediums.

People suffering from diabetes and respiratory related problems should not eat potatoes, lady fingers [Okra] and beetroot.

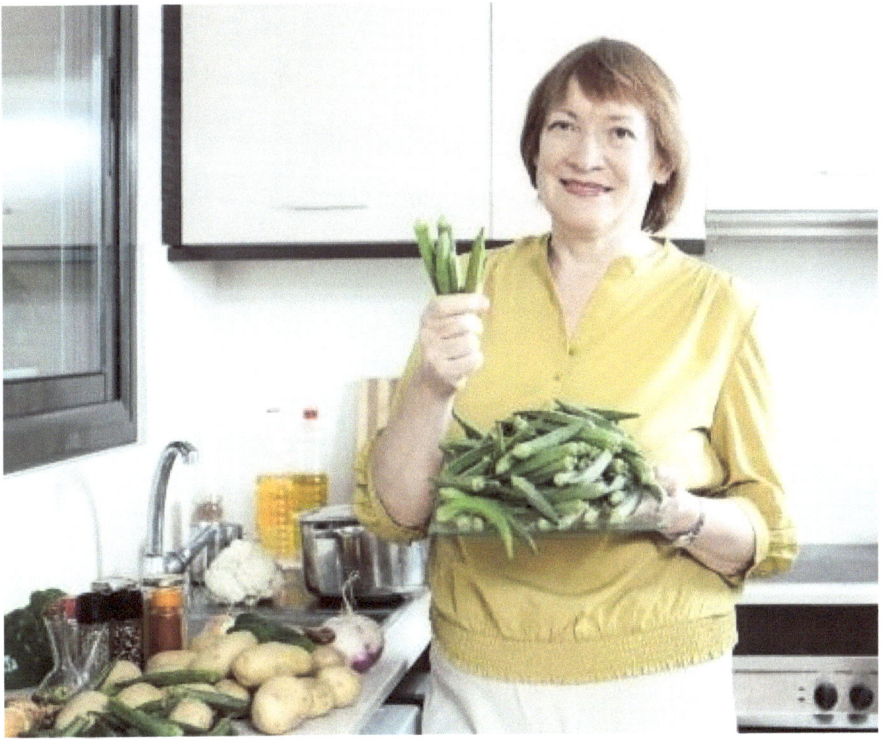

Excellent nutritional green, but definitely not for diabetics and asthmatics. So no gumbo and no okra fried with potatoes.

All right, this was something I found just by chance. I used to take out fresh tomato, spinach, radish and carrot juice, mix them all together, and drink down in one giant effort. That kept my system toned, because the juices were easily digested and assimilated in my system. One day I left this mixture in the fridge, intending to drink it with lunch. And I found myself suffering from flatulence. How come, and what had happened?

That was because instead of drinking these juices when fresh, I had allowed them to get stale for about four hours. So the next time you blend vegetables in your blender, for juice, drink it up immediately, with a little bit of lemon, rock salt and pepper to make it more palatable.

Do not ever cook tomatoes in copper pans. They are best cooked in stainless steel cooking pans. The best idea is to stir fry them in Woks.

Preserving Tomatoes after the Harvest Is in

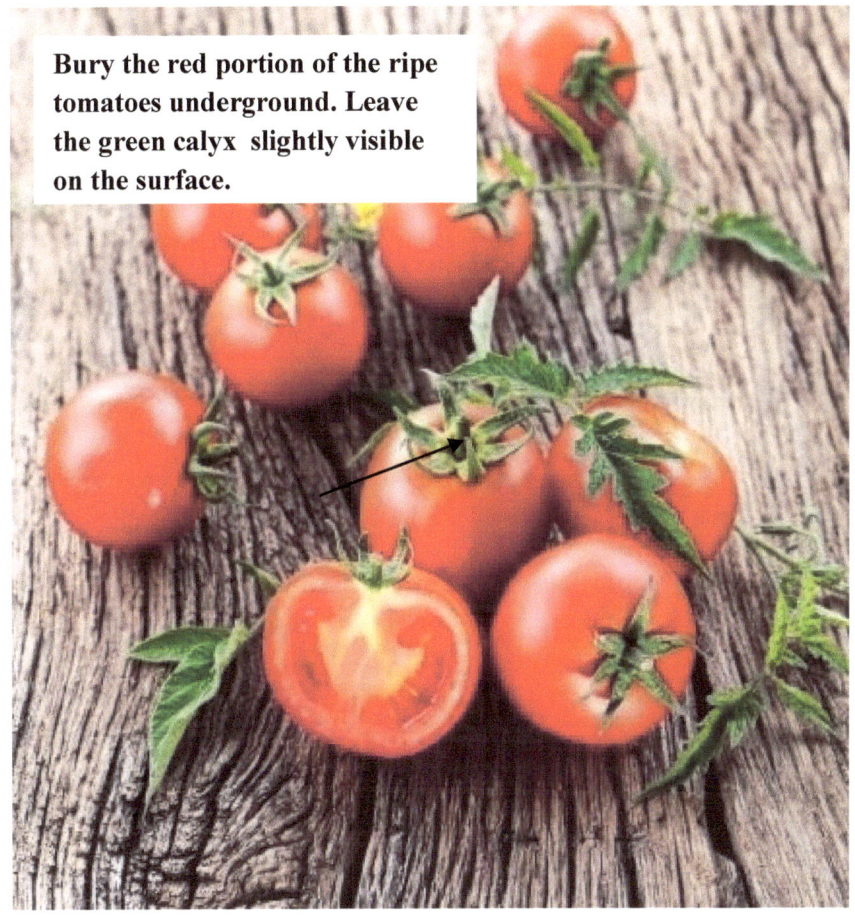

Bury the red portion of the ripe tomatoes underground. Leave the green calyx slightly visible on the surface.

Try preserving tomatoes by burying them – green stalk up – in a garden bed.

This is something which I saw in a very rural village, – no refrigerators around – where a tomato harvest was preserved by getting in the tomato crop and **not** removing the green stalk. Then a hole was dug in the garden, and all the tomatoes were placed stalk side up in the garden bed. So any time anybody wanted fresh tomatoes, she just went and pulled up a tomato from its preservation burial site. Ingenious, I must say.

Getting Rid of Mustard Taste

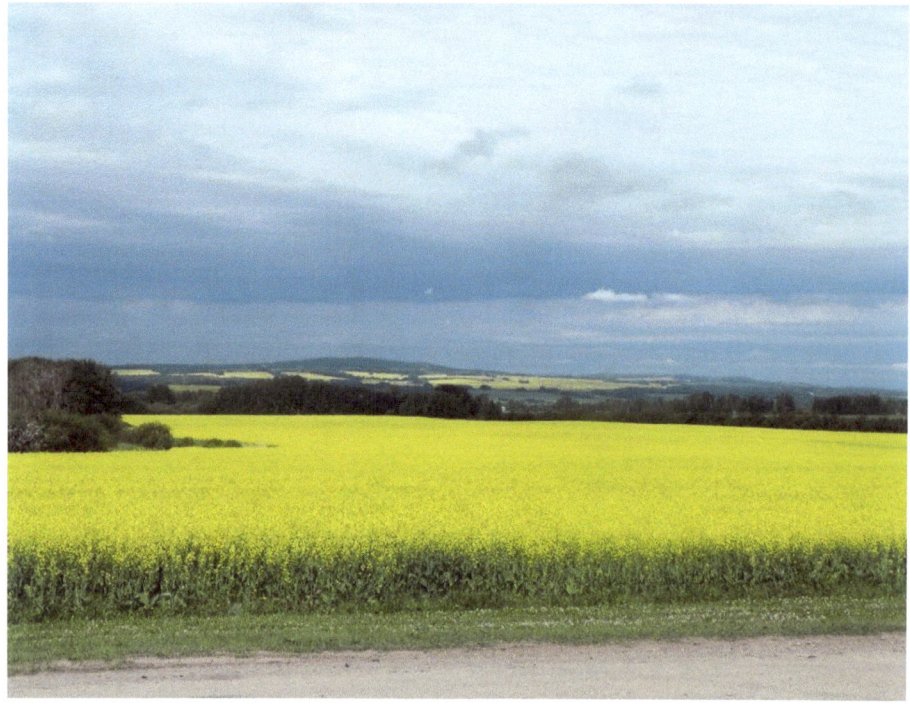

Mustard is a delicious green when eaten with butter, green chilies, raw onions and cream and when cooked well.

This is another tip I learned from her. Green leafy mustard is very popular in the Northern part of the Indian subcontinent. But it is an acquired taste, just because it tastes, well, mustardy and strong. Also, cooked mustard is slightly bitter after it has been cooked. So the moment she cooked it, and was preparing it for garnishing and ready to serve, she dashed one cup of icy cold water over that mustard. After that, she gave it a little bit more of heat treatment, so that the water was incorporated in the mashed vegetable leaves.

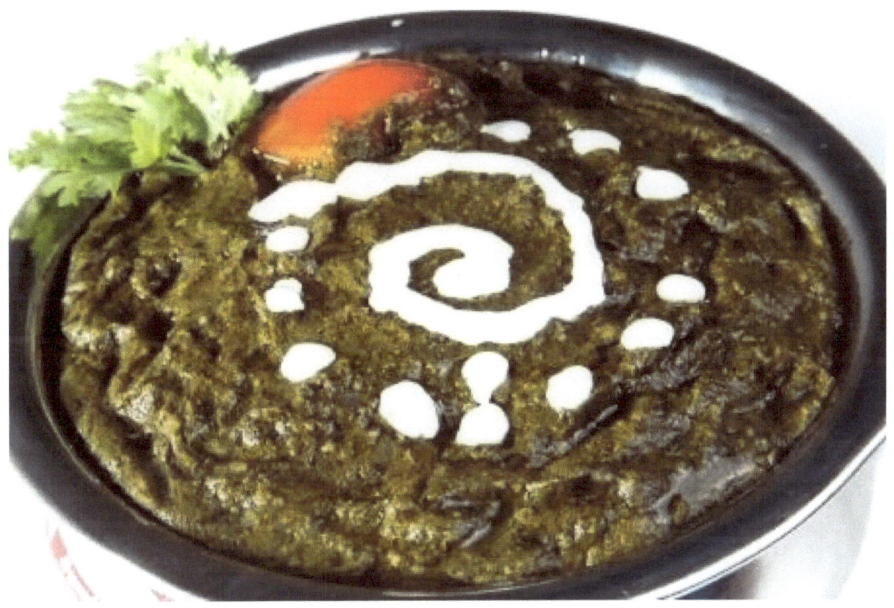

She then served it with raw onions, green chilies and a chunk of white homemade butter or cream with cornbread. This is the staple diet of the North Indians.

Boiling Old Potatoes

This is a tip which I caught from a farmer who had broken into his previous year's crop of potatoes. He knew that boiling them would leave some portions of them raw from inside. So he added a pinch of sugar and half a teaspoonful of lemon juice to the boiling water and then put the potatoes to boil. Hurray, perfectly boiled potatoes.

Curing Baldness with Cucumber

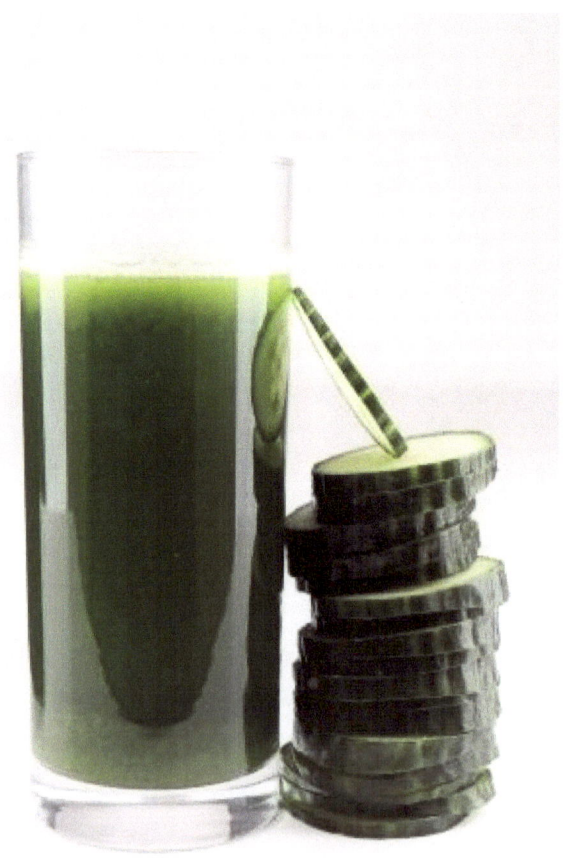

Drink this cucumber juice, as well as apply the juice and the pulp on your scalp for 15 days. If you do not suffer from a hereditary proneness to baldness, you are going to see your hair growing again. It works.

Hair Fall

In the same way, if you are suffering from hair fall, apply cucumber pulp or cucumber juice to the scalp. Keep it on for one hour and then shampoo your hair. This strengthens the roots of your hair and promotes its growth.

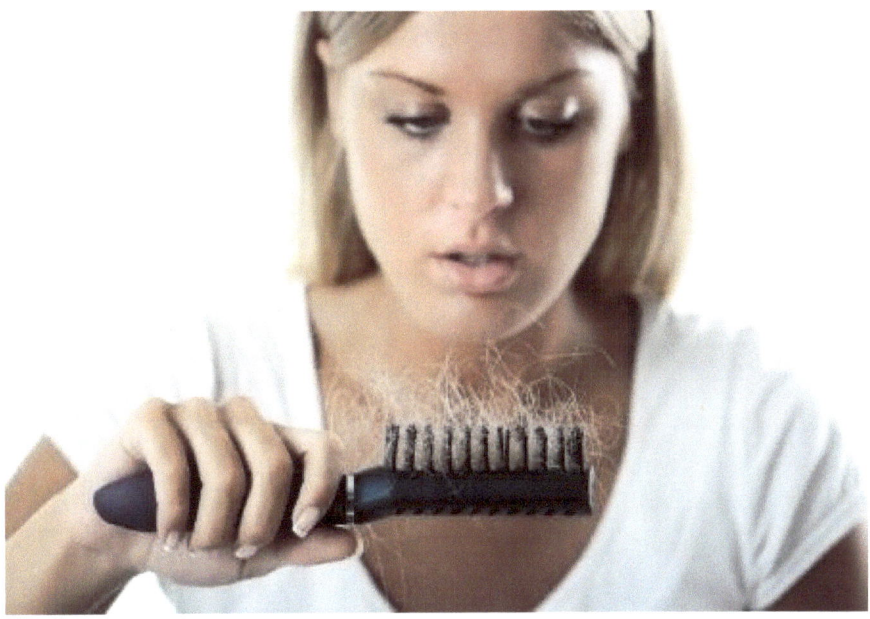

Curing Acidity

This is a time tested remedy, which you can try if you are suffering from acidity.

Eating unpeeled cucumbers without salt is going to cure you. On the other hand, if you eat cucumbers salted and then eat a heavy lunch over the salted cucumber, you are going to suffer from acidity, thanks to the food ingested.

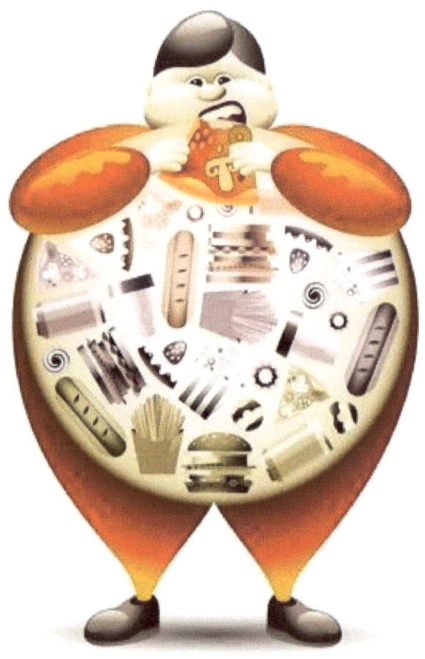

Acidity and other digestive problems are going to occur, if you eat rich and fatty food indiscriminately.

Rather amusing. That is why since ancient times, people were asked not to drink water after they had their meals, but they had to finish up a salad of cucumber, tomatoes and raw onions, – onions in the summer, – and unsalted.

Fenugreek Leaves and Seeds

Fenugreek has been known since ancient times as the best healthy medicine, both in its leafy form and in its spicy form in the shape of fenugreek seeds. You can make a mixture of spinach and tomatoes with fenugreek in a delicious dish. This cleans up your digestive system, keeps your system, warm, and that is the reason why it is eaten so much in the winter, and also, is considered to be the best internal skin tonic in the East.

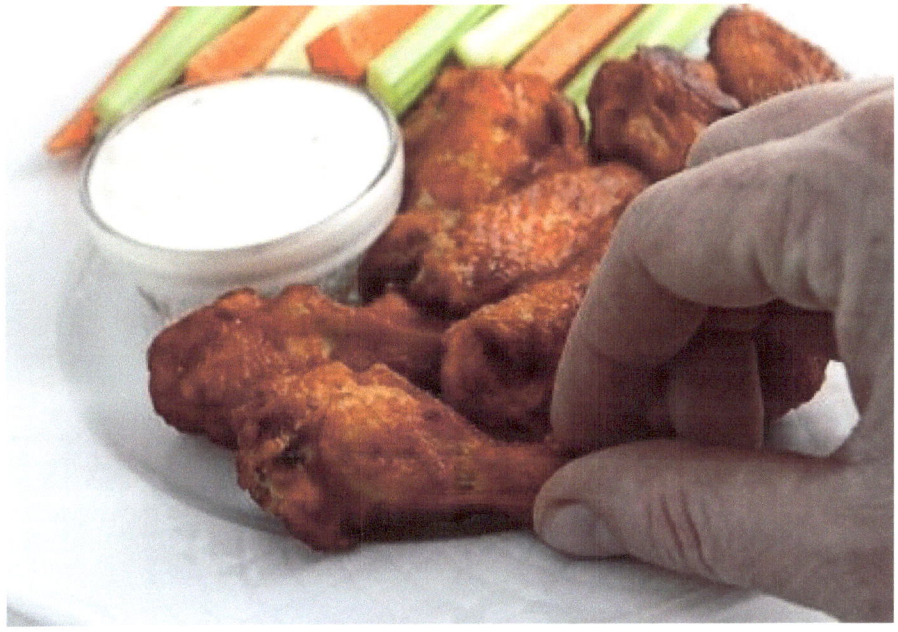

I am certain fenugreek seeds were a part of the spices used in the marinade of this protein rich, hard to digest fried chicken.

Many enterprising farmers make sure that they raise a crop of fenugreek, before sowing a harvest crop, because this is going to add to the nutritional value of the soil. Try it out, if you are a farmer.

Fenugreek is good for people suffering from a low libido and anemia, thanks to its iron, sulfur and manganese content.

Do you find some foods hard to digest? Just add roasted fenugreek seeds to the gravy. It is also thought to be a good way in which you can lose fat. Add soya and fenugreek seeds to anything which you consider hard to digest. In fact, protein rich foods always have some fenugreek seeds added to the spices. That means the eaters are not going to suffer from heartburn, acidity and other digestion related problems.

Getting Rid of Jaundice

This remedy normally was used in ancient times when nobody knew all about scientifically advanced ways in which to cure jaundice. Jaundice normally occurs when your liver is not functioning properly. Your skin turns yellow, because of a problem in the body's biliary system. Janice was treated by taking 30 g each of radish juice and radish leaves juice, mixing together with brown sugar and fed to the patient on an empty stomach, for 20 to 25 days.

Now, let me give you the scientific basis for this cure. The ingredient, which cure is the brown sugar. [And I am not talking the drug cartel here!] It is made up of concentrated Sugarcane juice. And everybody knows that Sugarcane juice is the best remedy to keep your liver healthy and happy. Also, in the summers, we were given lots of sugarcane juice to drink, so that our systems were well toned, and we never suffered from liver problems, even in areas where jaundice was very prevalent. Do not eat anything sour, while undergoing this treatment.

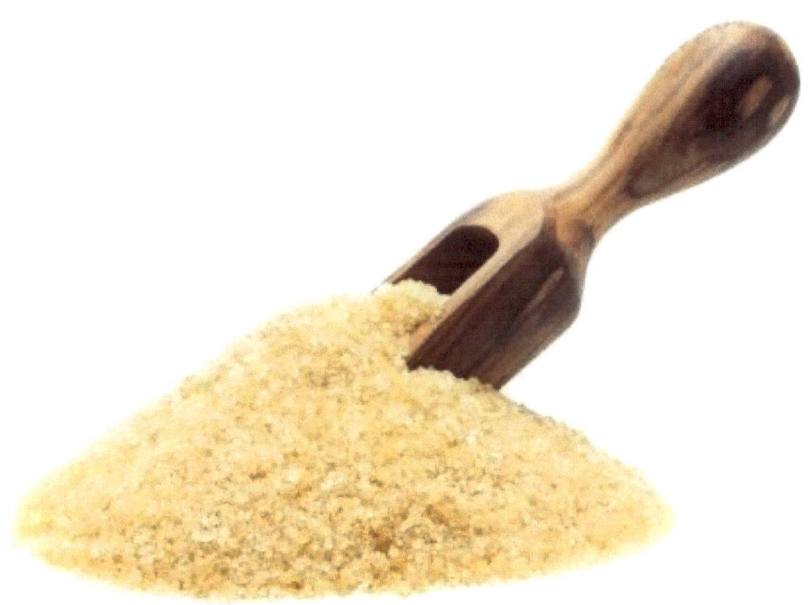

Organic Brown Sugar

You may find this URL very interesting, to know how it is made in the Indian subcontinent.

http://www.youtube.com/watch?v=--NL7diaFdI

[Yes, it does look unhygienic, does not it. But I could not find a video with the process being made in more salubrious conditions.]

Of course, in Europe, it is made of sugar beet. This is called shakkar in the East. It is unrefined sugar and is definitely not going to be white in color. It also does not have any whitening chemical products put in it, and is very strong in taste.

Getting Rid of Migraine with Carrots

Migraine normally occurs, when you are suffering from tension, stress, or from food allergies. My migraine attacks were normally triggered off, when I was confronted with camera flash bulbs flashing! So lately tell you something about migraine. Women are more prone to it. This ailment, however, is going to peter off when they reach their 40s and 50s, unless there is something drastically wrong with their system. I have not had a migraine attack for the last 10 years, though I used to suffer from it continuously when young. And it could be brought about by the stupidest reasons like eating chocolate, being stressed, low blood pressure, or anything else you could think.

And this is the migraine remedy, which I used to apply, when I did not have a tablet of Vasograin around. Lie still in the dark bedroom and pray for sleep. As I did not take any sleeping tablets then or now, I did not resort to artificial drugs to put me to sleep. I used to suck on a salted lemon to prevent nausea. And my grandmother crushed some carrot leaves and trickled the warmed juice into my nostrils and into my ear, every 15 minutes. It worked for me because the attack disappeared by the next morning.

I really do not know the scientific explanation for this. But I suggest that as you have a different biochemical metabolism, if you suffer from migraine, you may want to take the shortest cut – a nausea preventer, and the migraine tablet recommended by your doctor. He may also prescribe some knockout drop. Why suffer pain stoically?

Tomatoes for More "Blood"

Eating lots of raw and unpeeled tomatoes is considered to be good for increasing RBC in your body.

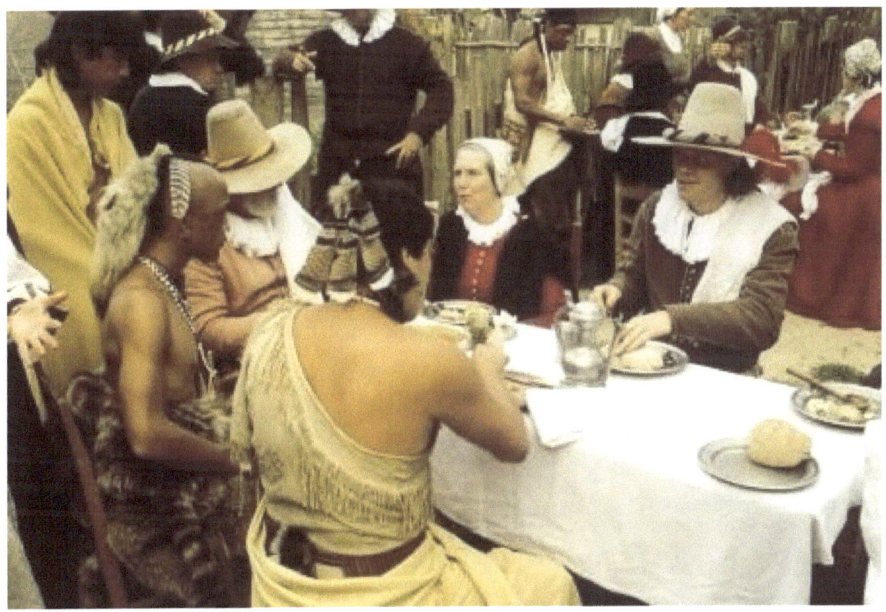

The first Thanksgiving harvest in Plymouth, Massachusetts was celebrated by the pioneers, with their Indian friends. This friendship and happy symbiotic relationship lasted for about a *hundred years* until the coming of people in the late 18th century onwards who did not want to colonize that land, but to conquer it and grab it from the original native indigent settlers.

Did you know that tomatoes, not being an indigenous berry in the East, was until late considered to be a taboo fruit, because it was blood red in color?

In fact, early pioneers and settlers in America also considered this fruit dangerous to eat, because they did not quite trust its color. And it was the red Indians, who, being very friendly with the colonists in the initial stages – until a Dutch governor decided to exterminate them, and introduced the idea of payment against every Native American scalp brought in. And so the Native Americans learned all about scalping, and are now notoriously associated with such a barbaric European practice – taught them about its nutritional value.

This story was told to me by a Lenape friend. It seems the mayor of New York, welcomed a visiting native Lenape Indian chief in the 1960s by showing him around Manhattan . The mayor could not resist saying, "How do you like my city?" "Very fine", said the dignified chief, "How do *you* like my country?"

The Lenapes were the original inhabitants of Manhattan. These Native American tribes were extremely versed in herbal lore and they knew all about the value of local indigenous fruits and vegetables.

Tomatoes have a high iron content. So eat them raw or in juice form. Remember to remove the seeds before drinking, because they have a tendency of aggravating stone problems, if you have any.

Juices for Blemishes and Black Spots

Is your skin suffering from blemishes, or black spots? Try a mixture of 50 g each of tomato [deseeded], carrot, beetroot and orange juice. Drink it regularly for about one month. This is going to get rid of all the pigmentation problems in your body. Extend this treatment for another month to get rid of blemishes, pimples and other skin ailments.

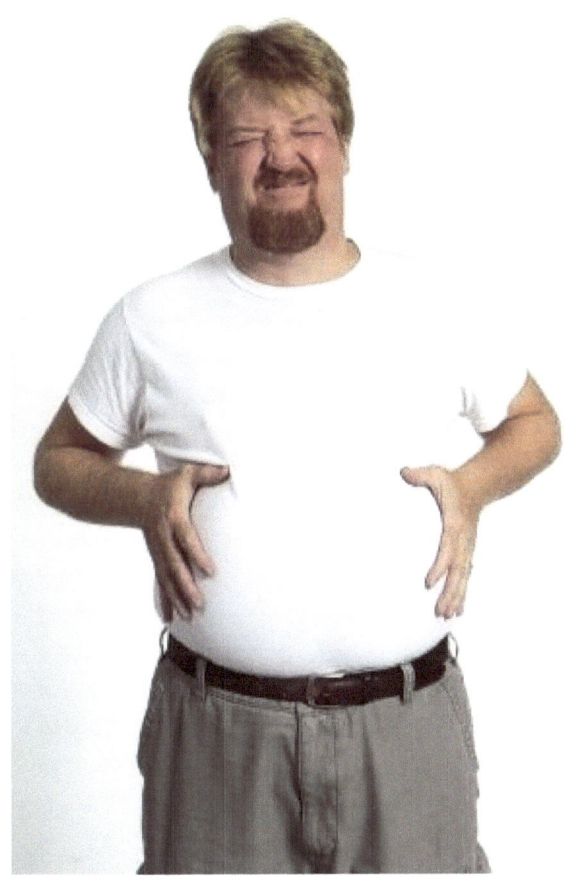

Tomato juice is also excellent to cure constipation.

Remember to eat just the pulp of a tomato, when you are eating it in salad in juice form or in raw form. The seeds often cause problems in your tummy.

Scars

If you have any scar marks on your body, which have not been caused through burns, these can be removed by extracting the pulp of a tomato and applying it on the affected area. Do this every night before sleeping, for one week. It takes one week for the healthy skin to start growing to the normal color of your skin.

Diabetes Cure

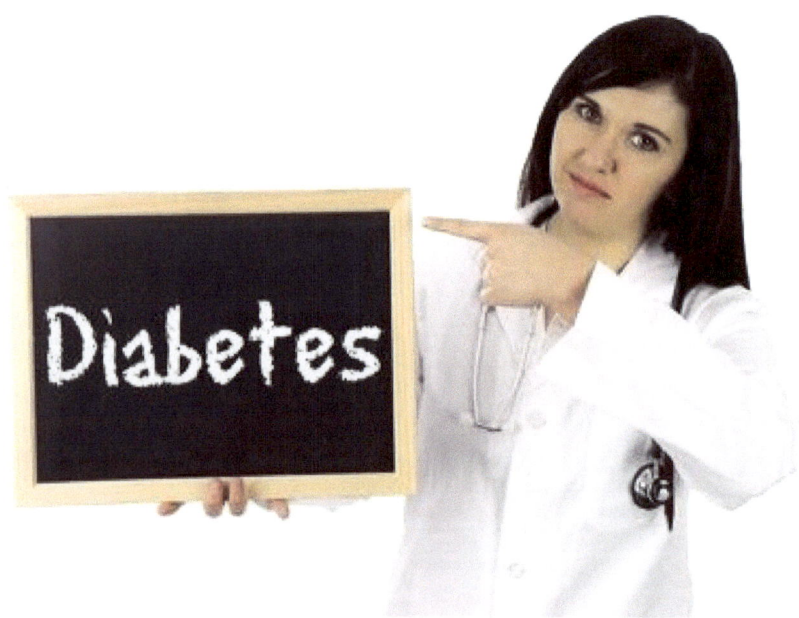

Now this is a remedy which researchers should look into. A Korean friend who learned it from her grandmother told this to me. Diabetes can be managed and often controlled with the help of turnips!

Turnips for Controlling Diabetes

Turnips are normally a winter vegetable, but if you have lots of turnips around, just sun-dry them, package them, and eat them throughout the year. Also, make a tomato soup, after you have deseeded the tomatoes.

Healthy Tomato Soup Recipe

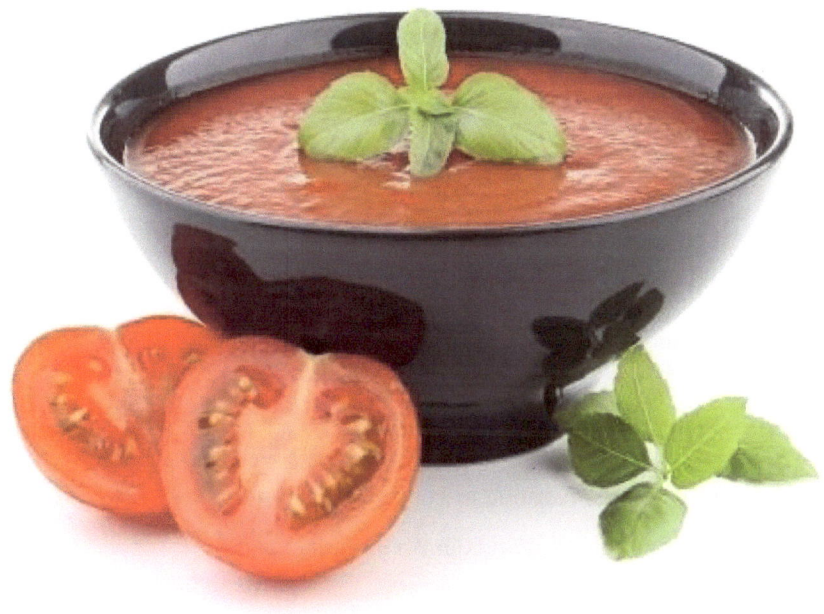

This is a traditional tomato soup, brought to you all the way from Provençale and for six hungry people.

You need one kilogram of fresh ripe tomatoes.

One large onion, minced

Three cloves of garlic crushed or just chopped into small pieces. [We are talking French traditional cuisine. So, we cannot do without garlic!]

One bay leaf

A pinch of thyme. The traditional original dish wants me to use the herb's flower, but I do not have it around

1 tablespoon full of castor sugar

2 tablespoons olive oil

Salt, pepper and cayenne pepper to taste

Cook the onion and garlic in the olive oil for two minutes and then add the tomatoes, salt, sugar, the bay leaf, the thyme , cayenne and pepper. Bring to a boil, and then lower the heat and allow this tomato soup to boil for 15 minutes.

Remove the bay leaf and then blend in a blender. Strain the soup and chop some basil for garnishing, and add some olive oil before serving. This is delicious in winter, when served hot, and also when served cold in summer.

Preventing Dehydration

Did you know that it is possible to get dehydrated in the winter too? We are so used to drinking lots of liquids in the summer, that we forget that our body needs lots of liquids throughout the year. But because it is cold in winter, we stop drinking those many liquids. That is why the find our skin getting dry and papery in the winter. We think that this is because of the cold, and apply moisturizing lotion and cream to moisturize the skin. But it is just our skin showing the first signs of dehydration.

Drink fresh tomato juice in morning and evening in the winter with a little bit of warm water added to it. In the same manner, if you find your skin getting really dry, add 10 g tomato juice to 20 g coconut oil or your favorite massage oil, like olive oil and rub the exposed skin with this mixture. Then bath in lukewarm water in half an hour. It is such a pleasure boiling oneself in hot water in winter, but that is the easiest way in which you can lose your body's natural moisturizing oils. So if you really want to soak yourself in a really hot bath every evening – just like I – remember to moisturize your skin afterwards with a bit of olive oil or coconut oil. Try not to use artificial moisturizers as far as possible. The tomato/oil remedy is going to get your skin well moisturized and silky, shiny in just two days.

Burn Cure

Now this is something which I saw being used by the native tribals in the jungles in which I lived. Fire was a necessary part of their lives, and so were burns, especially in forest fires. That is why they always had grated potatoes with them. The moment they got burned, they just slapped on the potatoes with potato juice on the burns. This took away that horrifying pain of burns in a while and helped cure the burns.

Now this is a time-tested native remedy, and I know that the burn scars can be lightened slowly and steadily with the application of a turmeric paste. But I suggest that if the person has been really badly burned, take him to a doctor immediately.

The native tribals – the friends of my childhood and youth – did not do that, because they knew nothing or could not be bothered about hospitals and doctors. But they did not mind the burns getting cured naturally, and they were physically strong enough not to worry about such trivialities.

This was an inconsequential part of their really hard lives, and I remember as a child, a tribal classmate -[*C. Kunkal, he was nicknamed Dark Horse, by our physical trainer and teacher, because one did not know that he was as fleet footed as an Arabian horse. That is when the rest of us ordinary mortals were sidelined as future prospective athletes and the tribals with their inherited physical, athletic qualities were inducted in all events and games. And they won them. We soon found that we could not compete against them. Just like the fleet footed Maasai, they were all Olympic level runners.*] - enthralling all of us – classmates and teachers – with stories about how his ancestors used to go trapping animals by just surrounding them, and tackling their legs just like one does in a football tackle to bring their opponent down.

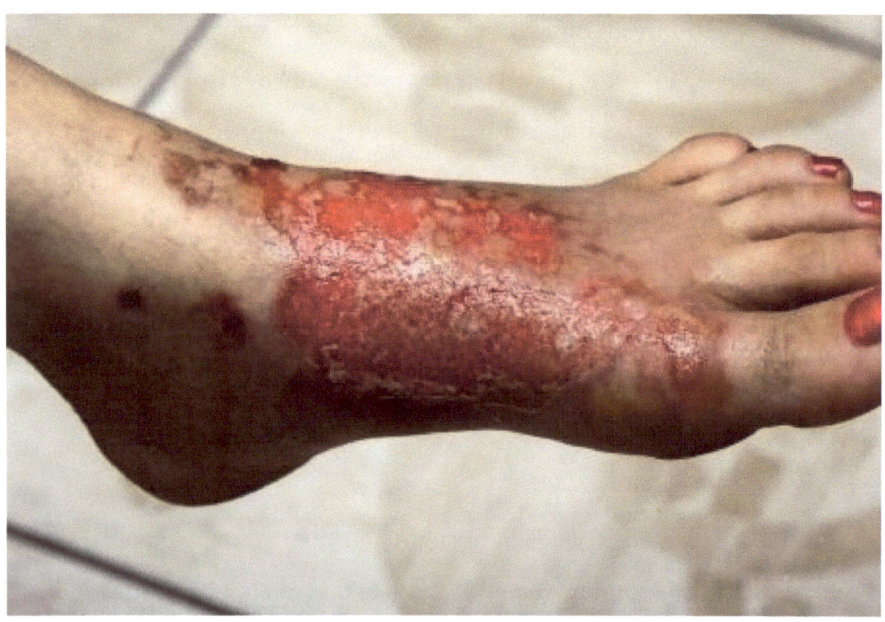

I remember us listening breathlessly to one of his stories told about his grandfather who thought that he was tackling a deer, but it turned out to be a bear. Naturally he got well clawed for his pains, until the rest of the team could come and kill the bear with their spears and arrows. Yes, this is a 20th century story.

And then grandfather got up, went to the river, and took out some mud from its bottom. He plastered it all over his open wounds to stop the bleeding and the whole tribe went singing back home, swinging the bear behind them. They would feast for the whole week on that delicious animal. Grandpa was 60 at that time, and a veteran of many hunts. He really came out of them unscathed.

As a matter of fact, bear meat is rather tasty, even if it is tough. Made the tribal way, it is beaten to tenderize it, before it is cooked in mud ovens, wrapped up in leaves and river Clay. The clay bakes the meat, and cooks it. Three hours in the coals and you have perfectly tender roast bear.

This is just an "airy persiflage" recipe. I do not know whether bear is still on the menus of a gourmet, but it was very much on the part of local native menus in the 40s and 50s.

Curing Heartburn

Many people are under the impression that heartburn is due to flatulence, or due to bad digestion. That is why they take flatulence remedies, which is temporary at best. I would suggest taking 2 tablespoons whole of raw potato juice, morning and evening. Do not add any salt to this juice. This is going to relieve you of that heartburn. Do not eat spicy food, including tomatoes, while you are getting rid of this problem in your tummy.

If you can manage to eat raw grated potato, without salt or spices, this is also going to help you a lot.

Curing Night Blindness

This is the night blindness cure, which was given to me by a tribal friend. They could not afford to lose their night vision, and so they made sure that they ate lots of wild tomatoes. They did not bother much about the seeds, but I have refined this process to make it more palatable to a more civilized palate. Collect ripe tomatoes, and deseed them. Then drink the juice. **Remember that the nutrients just below the skin are full of vitamins, so do not peel them at all.** Now, eat the pulp of the tomato without any salt or spices. This is going to get rid of any vitamin a deficiency in your body, and also take care of your night blindness. Try drinking fresh carrot juice also as a supporting supplement. You are soon going to see your night vision coming back.

Tomato – Potato Mix

In the East, obesity is a thing to be desired, because genetically, and traditionally, many of the countries were poverty-stricken, and people did not have enough food. That is why mothers fed their children this starch food in order to give them a well fed. Look. If you are already fat, do not eat this traditional dish. If you just want to put on a little weight, you can eat this twice a week.

Take the pulp of one tomato, and boil three potatoes. Fry them lightly together with rock salt, black pepper, and lemon juice. Feed with roti to a kid who seems to be losing weight due to a vitamin and carbohydrate deficiency.

Also increase the green leafy vegetable intake of your kid.

This mixture of potatoes and tomatoes can be made into pancakes and roasted on griddles. Then it is eaten with mint chutney. This is popular street food and is known as *chaat*-literally Lick,- and it is addictive and finger licking good. When made in hygienic conditions right in your kitchen, it is a very healthy meal because it has vegetables, yogurt and tasty , healthy spices. It is a vegetarian dish.

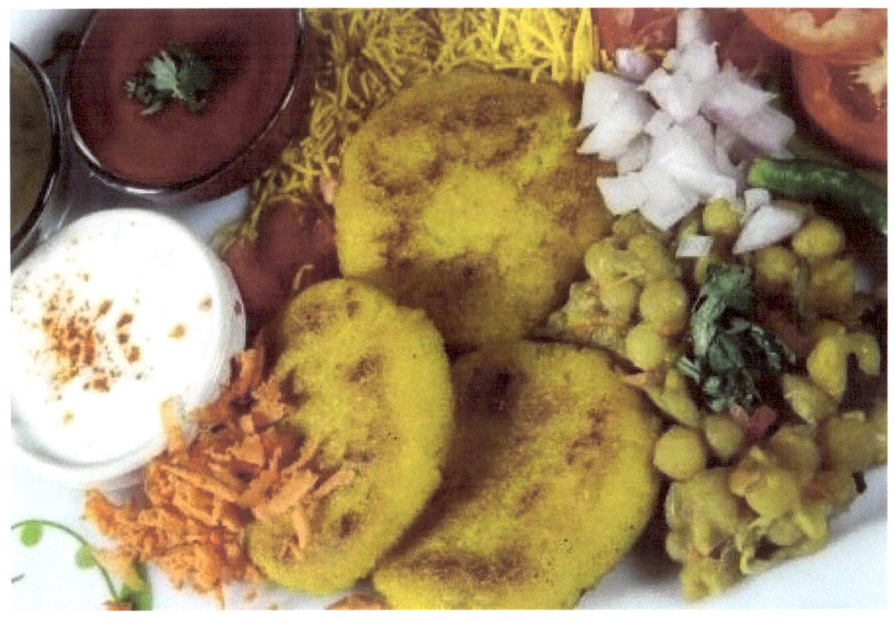

You can see chickpeas, grated carrots and onions, along with tomatoes, yogurt and mint chutney in this supposed street food, which is normally eaten, for tea.

Getting Rid of Headaches

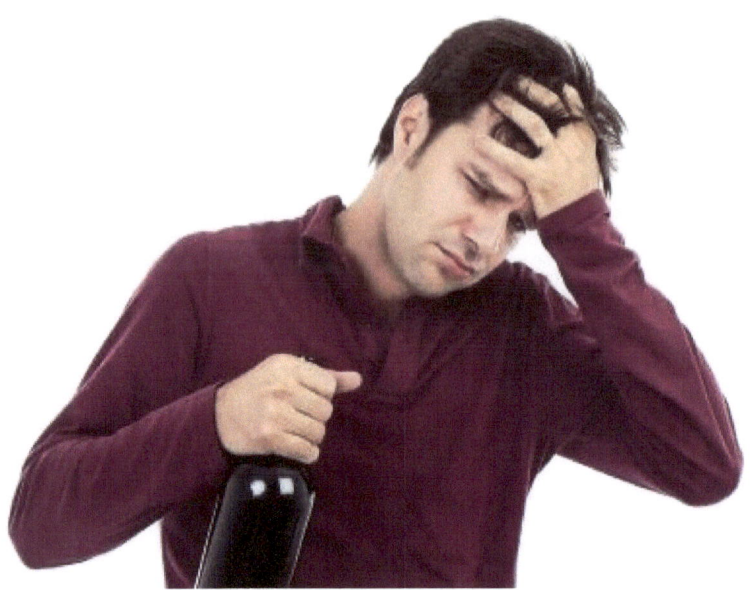

What brought this headache on? Dehydration can also cause headaches, especially when you have been drinking large amounts of alcohol.

This remedy has nothing to do with vegetables, but it has everything to do with getting rid of headaches the natural way!

Sugar Syrup

Have you tried drinking sugar syrup to get rid of headaches? I was extremely astonished to know that this was one of the ways in which headaches could be cured. Make a syrup of 6 tablespoons full of sugar in half a cup of water and manage to gulp down. That is only if you do not suffer from diabetes.

Black Pepper Decoction

You could also try a decoction of black pepper. Boil 12 powdered peppercorns in a cup of hot water, until you have half the amount of water left. Drink that down. I do not know whether it is autosuggestion, but I found my tension headaches disappearing after I had this powerful decoction.

If I was in a native Eastern or Northern village, I would immediately be sat down in the sun and my head massaged with a mixture of cold water, mustard oil and clarified butter. Two items highly pungent in odour. Lucky I am not in a village, even though this remedy is guaranteed effective. I guess, the powerful, mustard oil hitting your sensitive skin is enough to scare away any namby-pamby headache.

Tuberculosis Cure

All right, this is the first time that I am talking about a natural remedy for a really serious disease – TB.

Till the beginning of the 20th century, TB was one of the great silent killer in the West and in the East. Those who could afford it, sent their family members to sanatoriums in the mountains. But the majority of its victims like Satine in Moulin Rouge coughed their lives out in harsh cold surroundings. This was not only a major part of supposedly normal life in the West; TB is also very prevalent in the East. It can be cured, now. But the patient will always find himself vulnerable to chest infections.

A child born in the mountains coughing away was considered to be a part of natural life in the 30s in India. They just thought that he was weak, because they did not know much about TB.

My father was one such child. He spent his childhood and youth as a "kid prone to weak lungs, that is why he keeps coughing all the time..." So he had a miserable and perpetually sick childhood and youth.

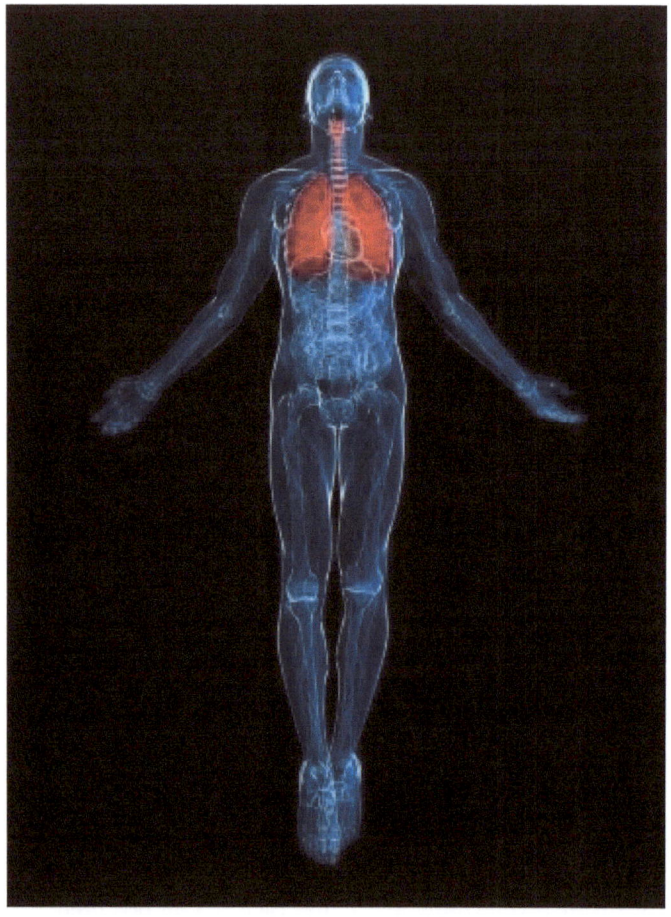

Fortunately, as an adult he spent six years in a dry desert area in Pilani Rajasthan, while learning to be an Electrical and Mechanical engineer. And that cured him of that pernicious cough, even though he has never gained a bit of weight till this day.

When he was a rather ailing student, his BITS Pilani doctors did not bother to tell him that he was suffering from TB. They called it possible pleurisy and cough. Being local doctors, I do not think they came across TB very often and could not diagnose it. They gave him cough medicines, which were just temporary reliefs. But Nature saved him.

He got to know all about his dreaded disease status, when he was in America in the 60s and the doctors at Carnegie Inst. of Technology *[now known as Carnegie -Mellon University of engineering. I think.]* Showed him the x-rays of his damaged lungs with scars still on them! And he had been cured completely, eight years previously, due to living in dry heat in the desert for six years! Who says nature is not the best healer?

He is now in his 80s and has never suffered from lung problems due to a *no visiting hospitals or visiting doctors, especially when in India* rule. He needed to get to America to get to know what was wrong with him!

Plenty of healthy food and plenty of healthy exercise, and also, I think good healthy genes keep him physically and mentally fit today. And also, he says that the only vegetable they got to eat in that benighted desert in the 50s were potatoes. Potatoes daily in some form or the other for six years, brought about a lifelong aversion to these vegetables in him. They did not fatten him. But the carbohydrates must have helped strengthen his system.

Cod Liver Oil Treatment

This is one cure, which he did not know, but which has come down the ages to cure tuberculosis. This was done by feeding the patient with the liver oil of sea fish with tomato juice. Remember that any available liver oil from any sea fish can do.

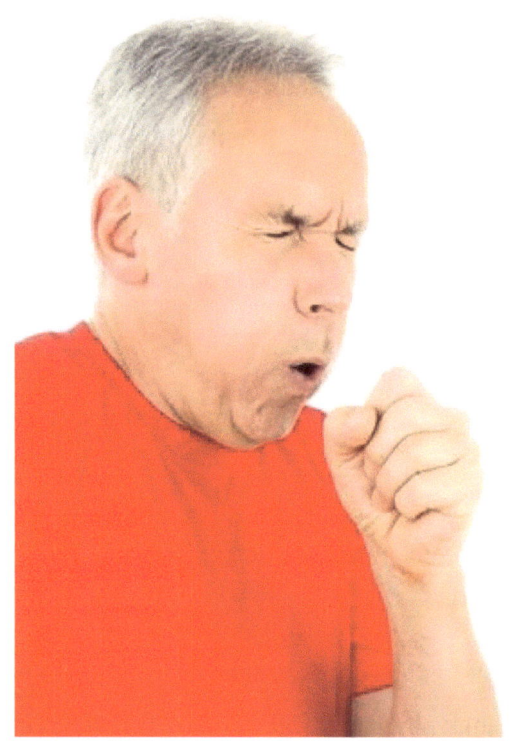

Cod liver oil is excellent for your body, especially when you reach your 60s and are prone to chest infections, including possible TB.

Aha, I told myself, when I heard this remedy. Cod liver oil! The ancients knew that it was very powerful, so they used to take 15 g of tomato pulp juice and mix it with hundred grams of liver oil juice. That means hundred grams of cod liver oil, verily and forsooth, because I have not heard about shark liver extract in my neck of the woods!

Ask the patient to pinch his nose and swallowing down, once a day. This treatment has to continue for **two months** without fail. The body is going to find itself healing within 1 ½ months, and you are going to see a visible improvement. But you do not stop right then. For the next one month you are going to feed him 7 g of seeded tomato juice in 50 g of cod liver oil once every day.

Then broadcast the results of he has been completely healed!

Get him to a dry climate, if you can. Cold Mountainous regions are not conducive to good and healthy lungs.

Conclusion

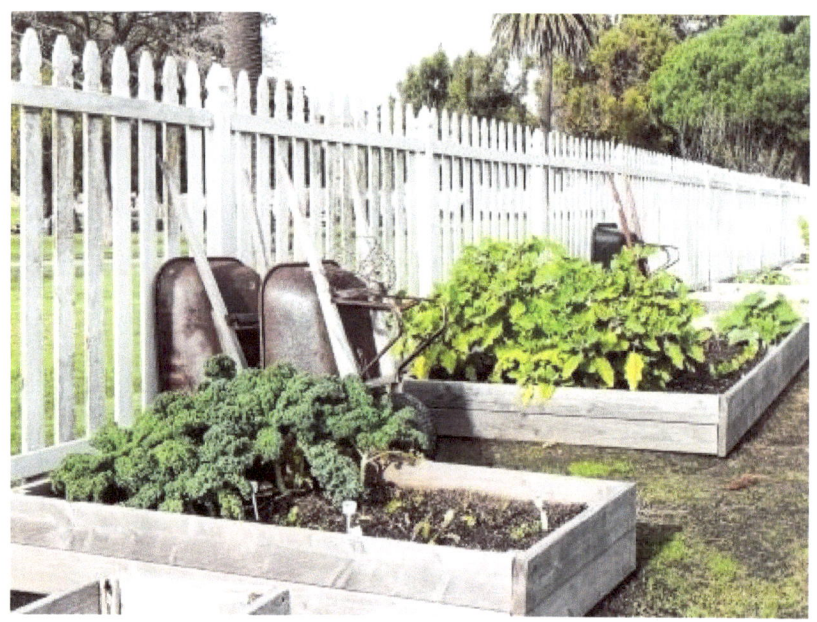

I hope you liked my book on vegetables and some tips. This is of course a mishmash of reminiscences, collected recipes, health remedies, experiences, and stories of my perpetually peripatetic and not so misspent youth, in areas where there were no doctors found very often, and one had to rely on nature and natural ancient herbal remedies and cures.

So since childhood, we were taught to eat our greens. And we stayed healthy.

We were also encouraged to eat fresh fruit and vegetables whenever we could, plucked fresh out of our gardens or pilfered from the gardens of our neighbors. Funnily enough, the stolen fruit tasted much better. And we considered one of these adults to be a real spoilsport.

He was the "Commanding Officer" of the project – the General Manager. And he threw his huge gardens, – fruit laden, and never mind that we had the same fruit in our own gardens – open to us, and told his security guard never to stop us from raiding his fruit trees and vegetable beds. As long as we ate them, and they benefited us, he was getting good Karma.

We immediately voted him "no fun!"

In fact, we told him that we had voted him "No Fun." And he said, smiling, "and here I was thinking that you would have enjoyed raiding my garden. Should I asked the guard to run after you when you are in the garden? He will enjoy doing that."

That, on contemplation was also considered "no fun". It was no fun – a guard, knowing that you were going to raid a garden, and just running after you perfunctorily and to amuse himself.

Growing up, I feel rather amazed about the deep insight into the psychology of a child by this very intelligent and nice gentle man, who unfortunately was childless. But then, he was also a bachelor so he was adopted as surrogate father by all the children, who showered him with lots of affection. He was so much better fun than all our parents who disciplined us regularly.

So his was the only garden left untouched. We particularly enjoyed raiding the gardens of the grouchiest Officers because it was such fun to hear them growl, "I am going to tell your daddy. Let him just come back from his office, just you wait. You are going to be spanked well, you thieving little brat."

Funnily enough, they never told tales to our parents, because they knew that their own children were away raiding somebody else's gardens and living life Emperor size. This was life in all its innocence and a healthy, happy childhood.

Look out for more books with ancient remedies, and reminiscences and stories in my magic series.

Keep well, keep healthy, and prosper.

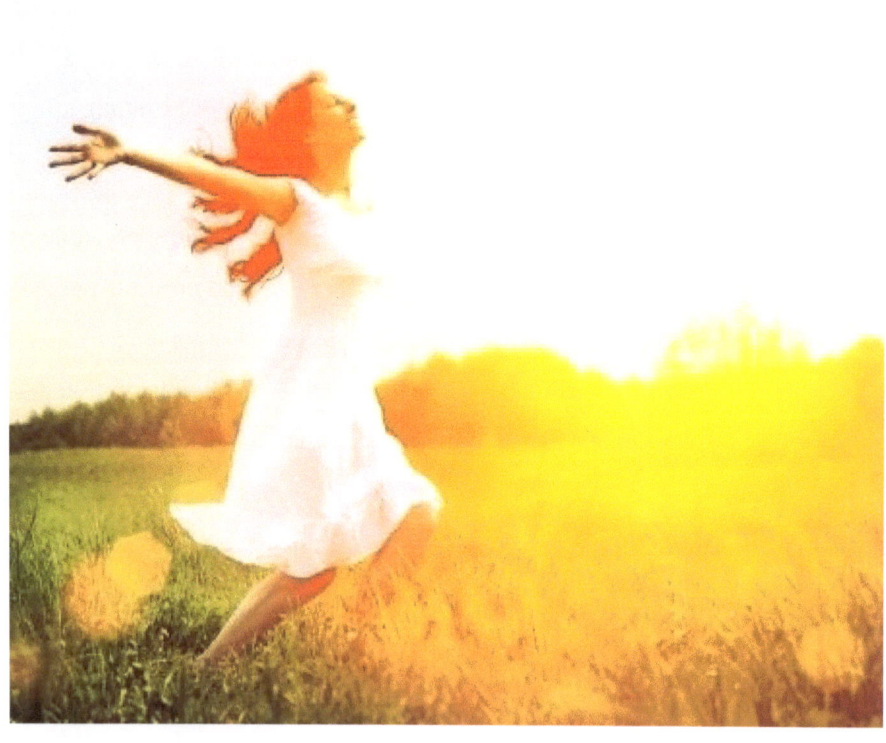

Author Bio

Dueep Jyot Singh is a Management and IT Professional who managed to gather Postgraduate qualifications in Management and English and Degrees in Science, French and Education while pursuing different enjoyable career options like being an hospital administrator, IT,SEO and HRD Database Manager/ trainer, movie scriptwriter, theatre artiste and public speaker, lecturer in French, Marketing and Advertising, ex-Editor of Hearts On Fire (now known as Solsctice) Books Missouri USA, advice columnist and cartoonist, publisher and Aviation School trainer, ex- moderator on Medico.in, banker, student councilor ,travelogue writer … among other things! One fine morning, she decided that she had enough of killing herself by Degrees and went back to her first love -- writing. It's more enjoyable! She already has 48 published academic and 14 fiction- in- different- genre books under her belt.

When she is not designing websites or making Graphic design illustrations for clients , she is browsing through old bookshops hunting for treasures, of which she has an enviable collection – including R.L. Stevenson, O.Henry, Dornford Yates, Maurice Walsh, C.N.Williamson, Sapper, Bartimeus and the crown of her collection- Dickens "The Old Curiosity Shop," and so on… Just call her "Renaissance Woman" - collecting herbal remedies, acting like Universal Helping Hand/Agony Aunt, or escaping to her dear mountains for a bit of exploring, collecting herbs and plants, and trekking.

Check out some of the other Health Learning Series books at Amazon.com

Health Learning Series on Amazon

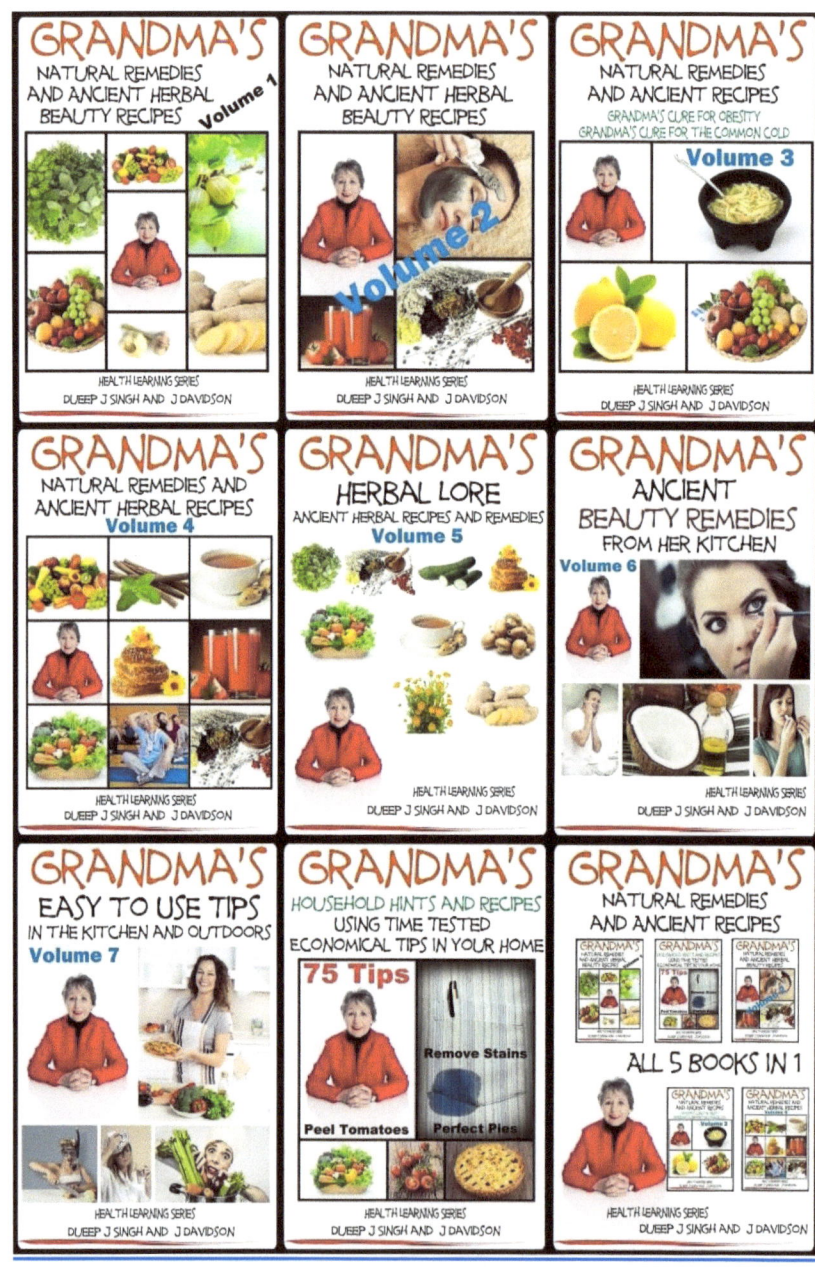

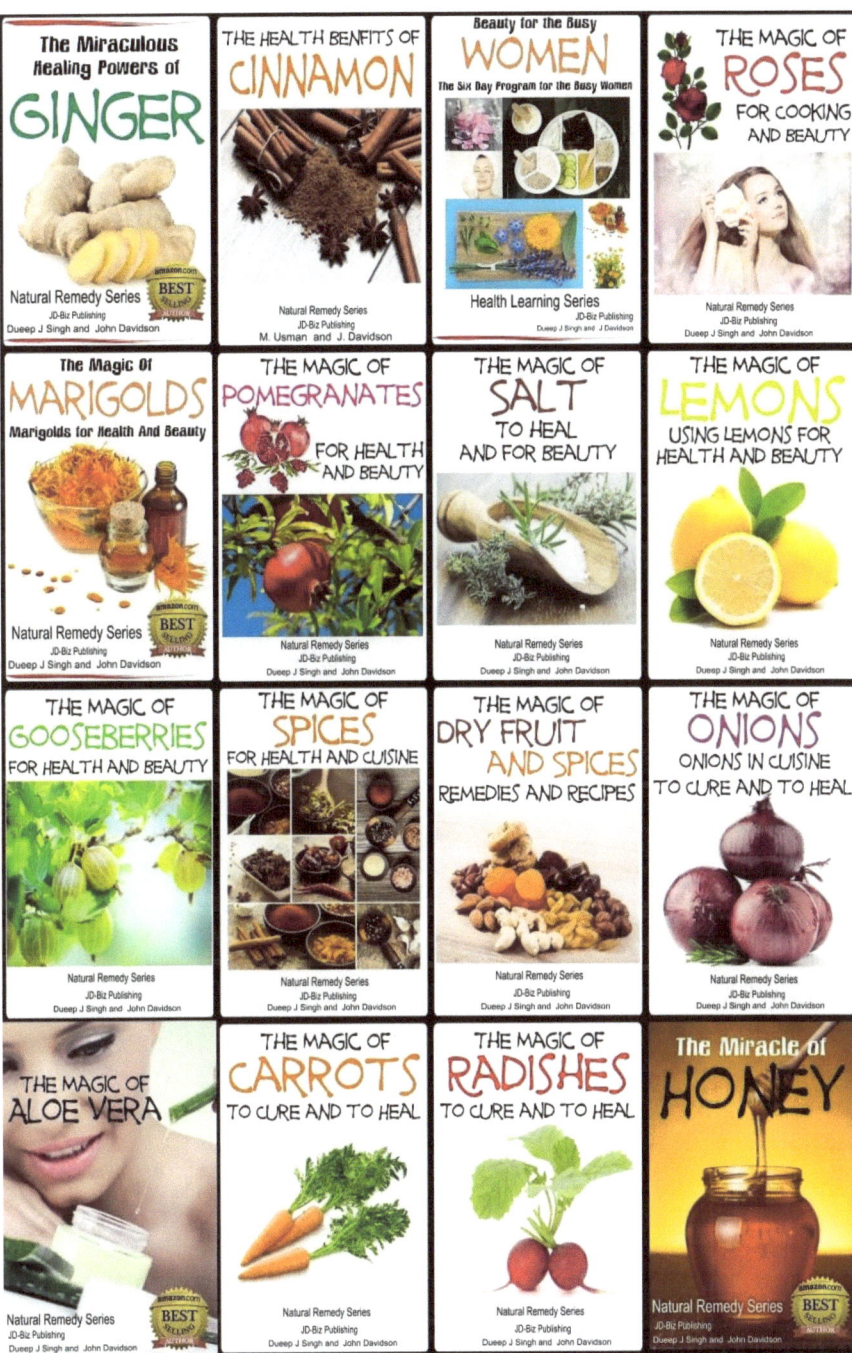

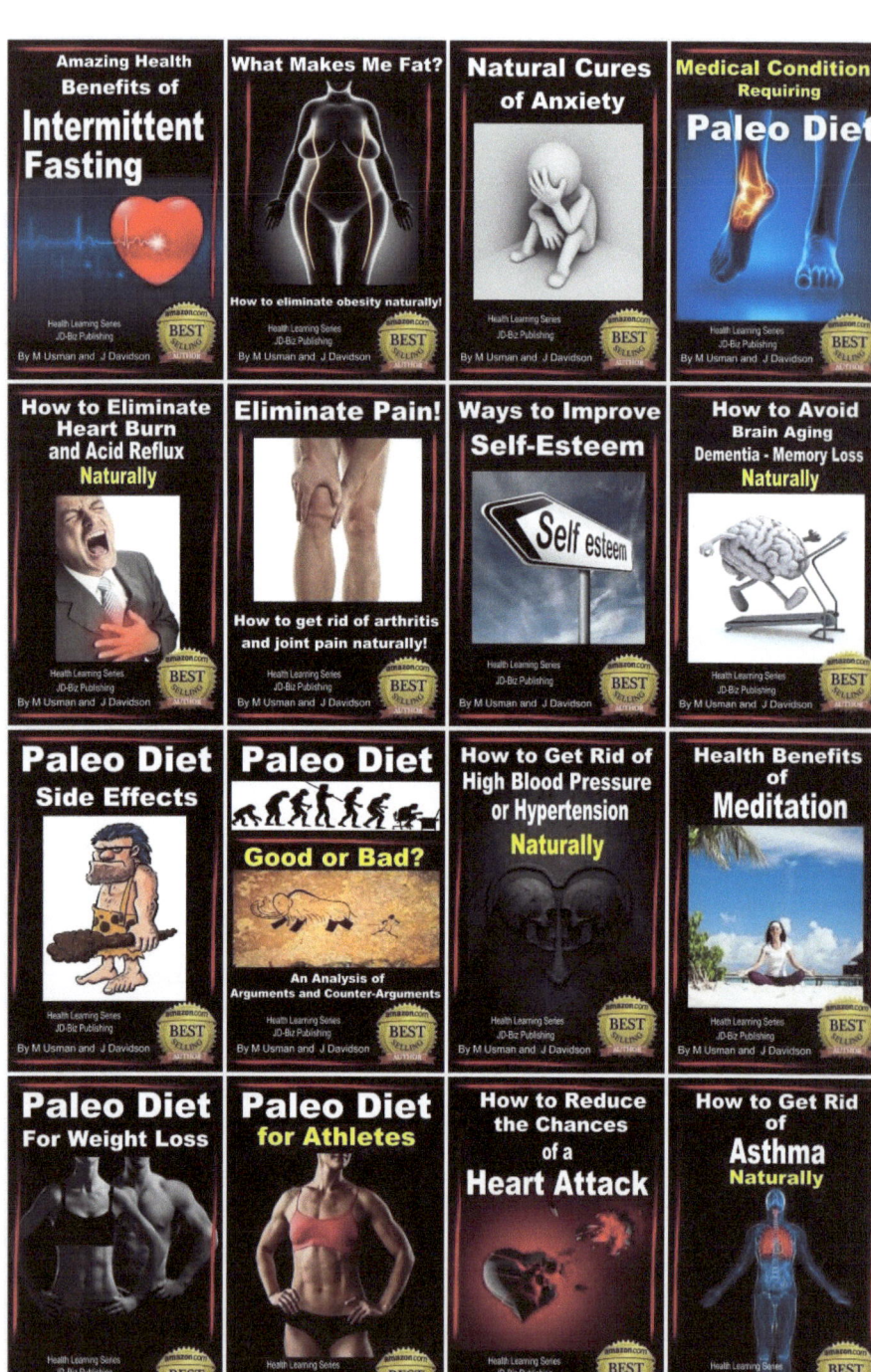

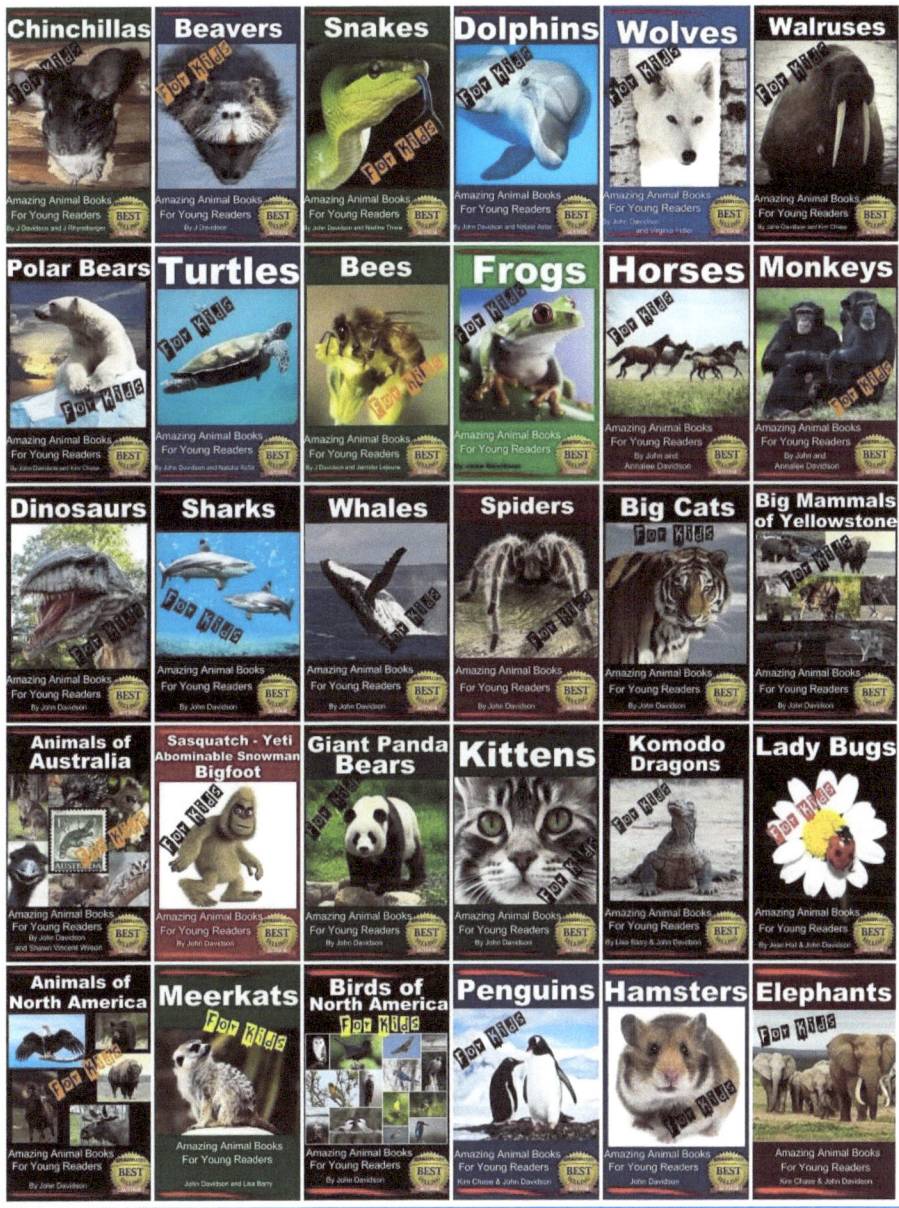

Learn To Draw Series

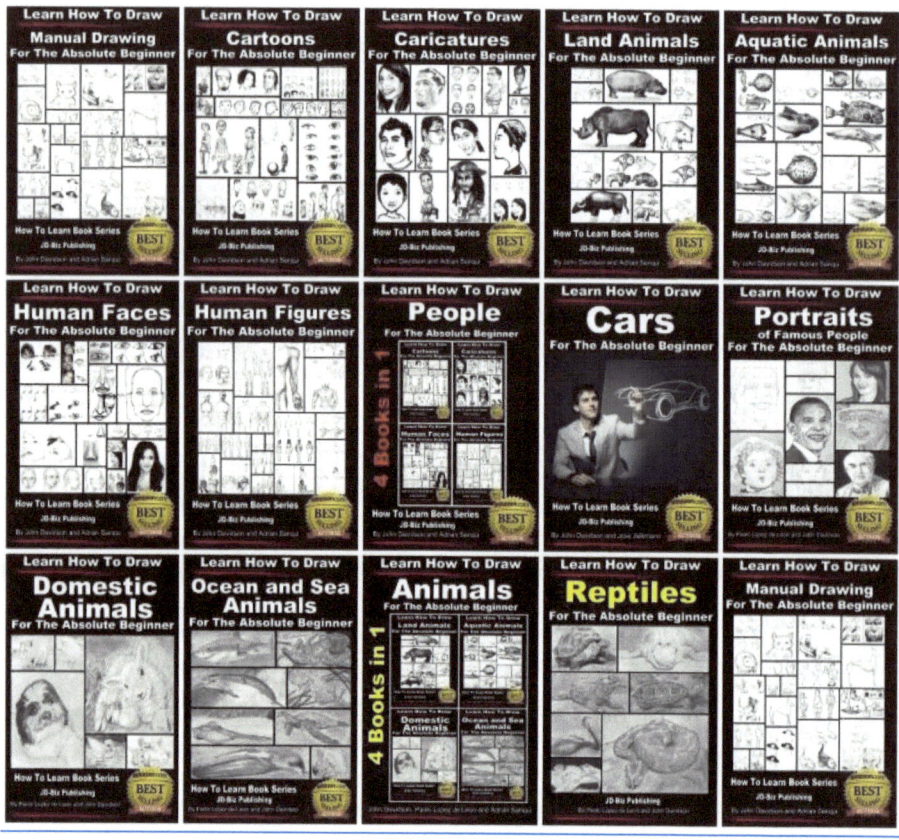

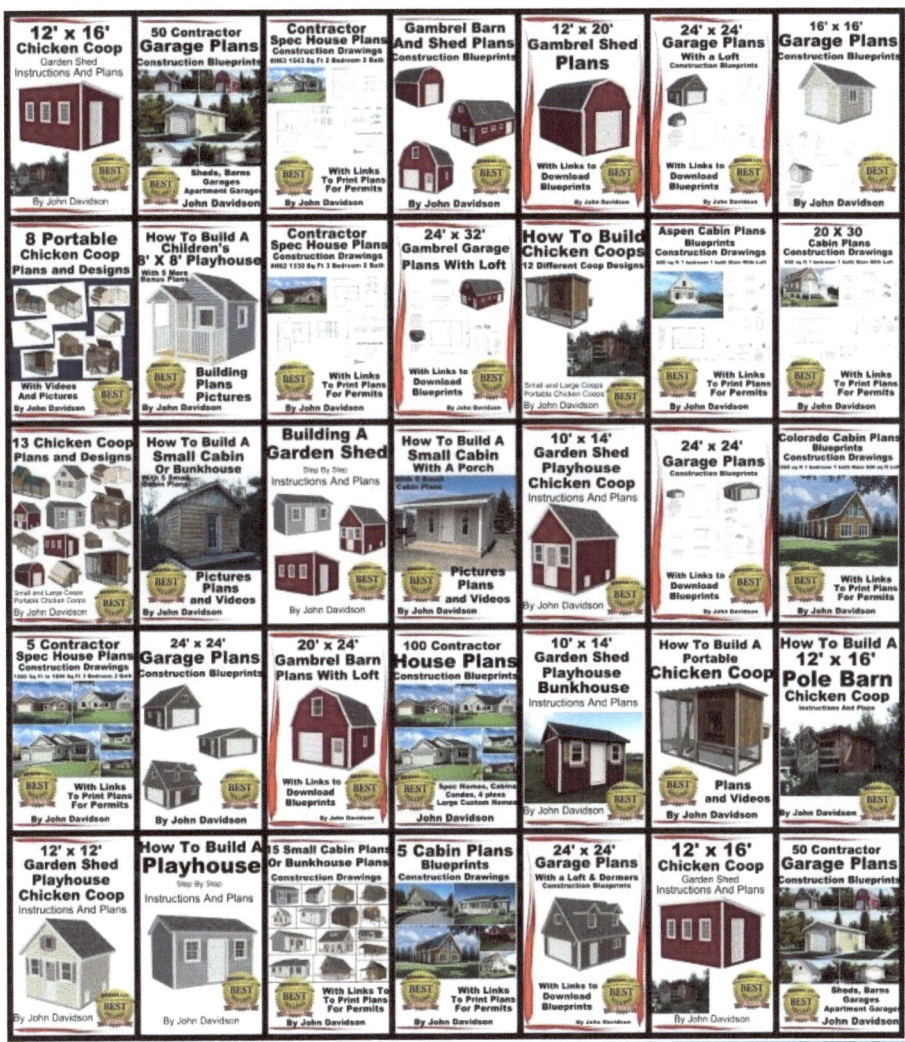

Our books are available at

1. Amazon.com

2. Barnes and Noble

3. Itunes

4. Kobo

5. Smashwords

6. Google Play Books

Download Free Books!

http://MendonCottageBooks.com

Publisher

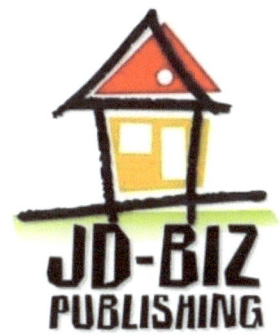

JD-Biz Corp

P O Box 374

Mendon, Utah 84325

http://www.jd-biz.com/

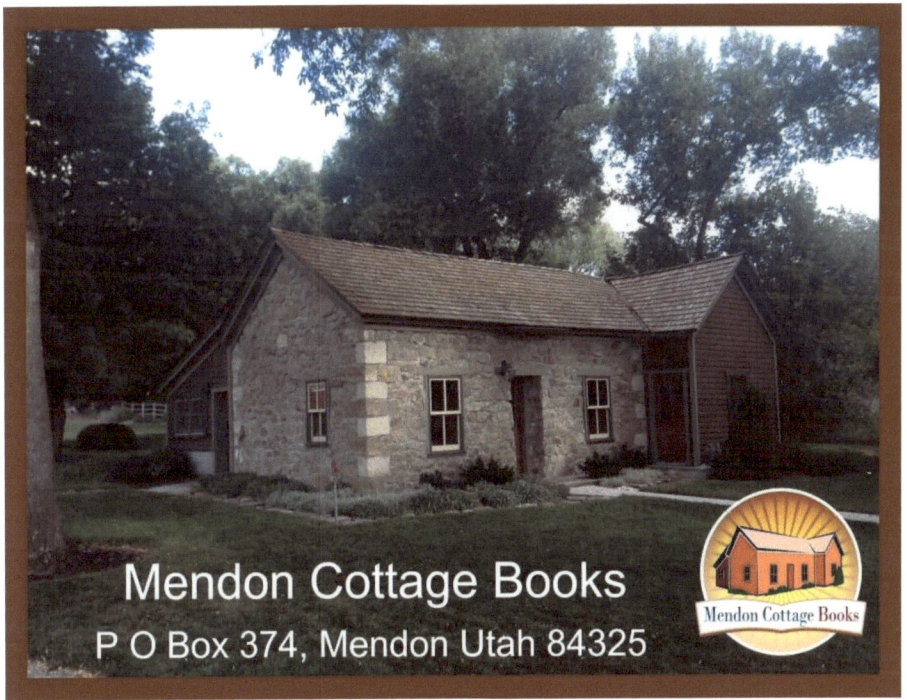

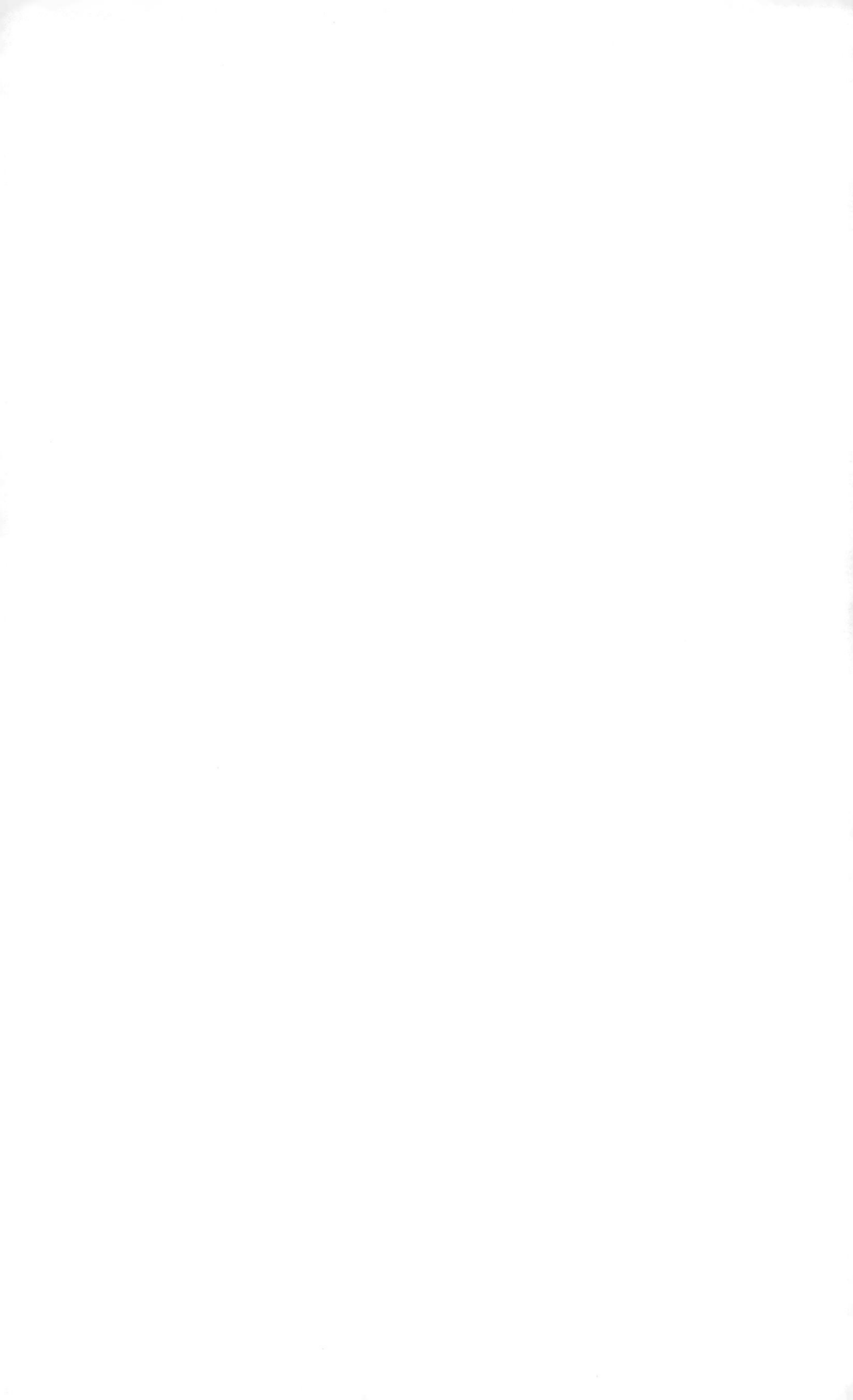

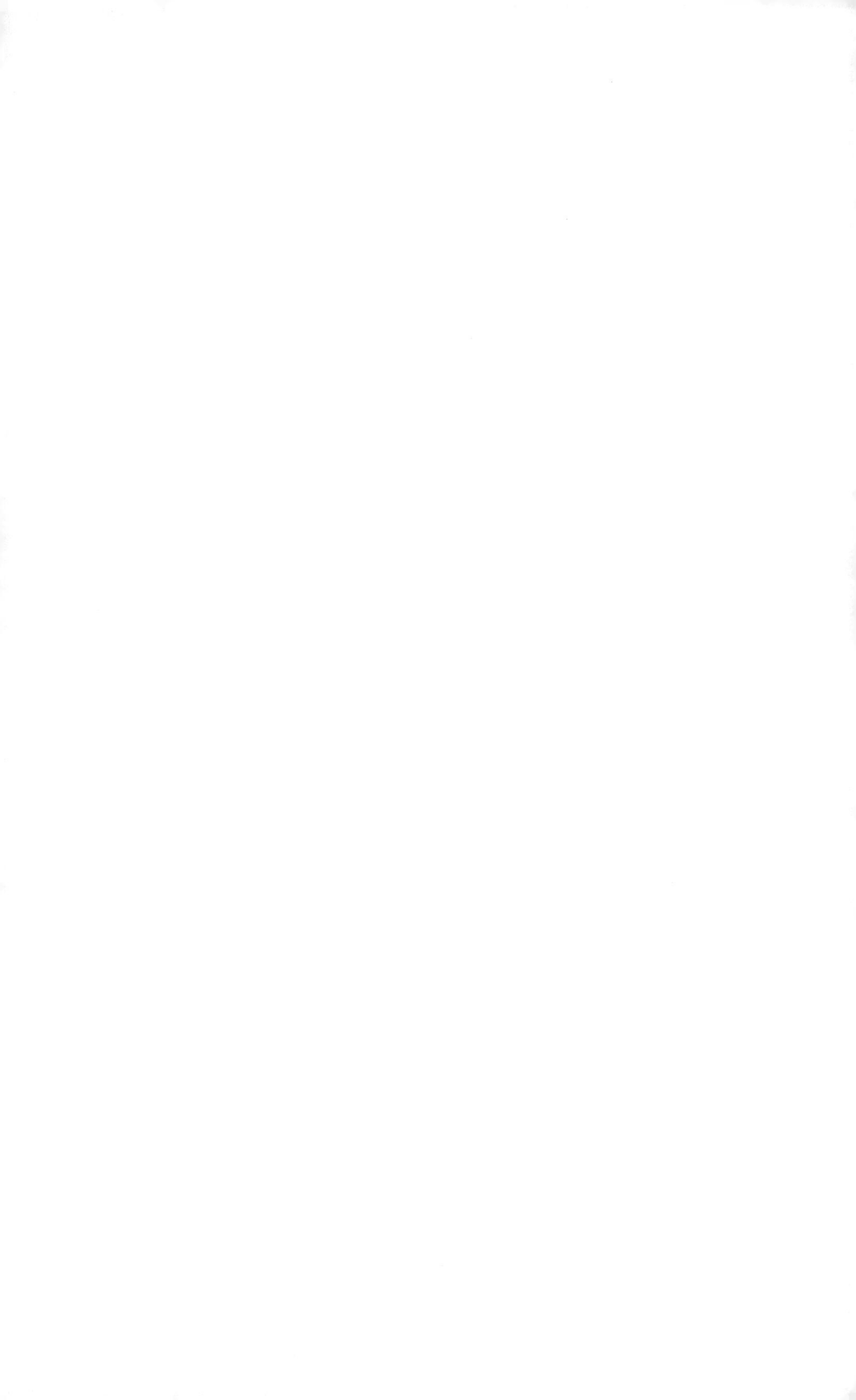

www.ingramcontent.com/pod-product-compliance
Lightning Source LLC
Chambersburg PA
CBHW050836290526
45792CB00001B/419